GRANDPA &

A story of hope and empowerment for children
touched by Lewy Body dementia

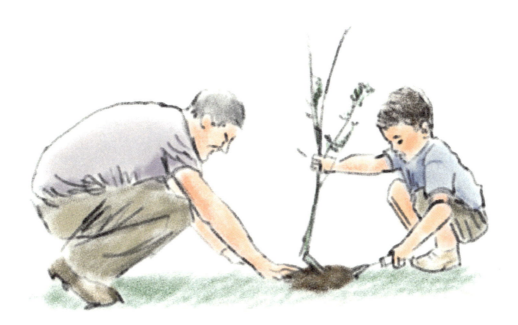

Jennifer Randazzo

As many as 1.4 million people suffer from Lewy Body dementia (LBD) in the United States alone, according to the Lewy Body Dementia Resource Center. Lewy Body dementia takes on similarities to the cognitive decline of Alzheimer's along with the impaired motor symptoms of Parkinson's disease wrapped up in one package that wreaks havoc on both the mind and body. When the cognitive impairment is heightened the person might experience better movement and strength. When the motor skills are affected the person may have lucid moments and an improved mental state. It was once explained to my family that the two disease processes were fighting for control of the brain. Lewy Body dementia is very difficult to diagnose and even more difficult to treat.

When my father was diagnosed with Lewy Body dementia fifteen years ago, we were initially told that he had two devastating diseases -- Parkinson's and Alzheimer's. He began to display cognitive, sleep and behavioral symptoms that eventually led to a diagnosis of Lewy Body dementia. Once we learned that it was Lewy Body dementia, we continued to refer to it as Alzheimer's and Parkinson's as no one had ever heard of Lewy Body dementia. For my dad, it was being stuck between two realities - one where the mind is lucid, but the body is failing you and the other where the body is strong, but the mind fails. The mind and body could no longer exist as a cohesive unit.

Well-known celebrities such as Robin Williams, Casey Kasem, and Sophia Petrillo are said to have suffered from Lewy Body dementia bringing more awareness in recent years. CNN Founder Ted Turner opened up about his struggle with LBD in a CBS interview in 2018. Even with this increased awareness--the fact that Lewy Body dementia is the second most common form of dementia, and in my opinion, the most devastating--most people still have never heard of it. My hope is that this book will not only help children who are faced with loving someone through Lewy; I hope that it will also help further raise awareness of Lewy Body dementia.

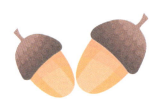

Copyright © 2020 by Jennifer Randazzo

All rights reserved. This book or any portion thereof may not be reproduced or used in any manner whatsoever without the express written permission of the publisher except for the use of brief quotations in a book review.

Printed in the United States of America

First Printing, 2021

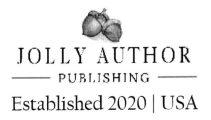

Established 2020 | USA

Dedication:

To my dad, whose faith never wavered even when Lewy Body dementia was taking everything he had. The kind of faith so strong that he knew God would not fail him – even on the darkest days. To my mom and all of the caregivers who give everything to care for a person that is only a shell of the person they once knew. To all of those affected by this disease and the long goodbye. You are not alone.

I can do all things through Christ who strengthens me. Philippians 4:13

Grandpa is my best friend. He knows all of my favorite games.
We love to laugh and play. He calls me silly names.
He loves to dance around and put on a funny show.
There's no one like my Grandpa. He is the grandest person I know.

We do lots of things together. We go for walks and have long talks.
We tell jokes. We laugh. We sing.

All I have to do is ask, my grandpa will do anything.
We love to lie in the grass and gaze up at the sky.
Looking for cool shapes as the clouds roll by.

At night he tucks me in and tells me a story. We talk about our
adventures that day. Grandpa always gives me an extra hug
before he turns to walk away. Whenever I have a bad dream Grandpa
tucks me in all over again and sends those scary monsters away.

I feel brave with Grandpa by my side. He always knows just what to say.

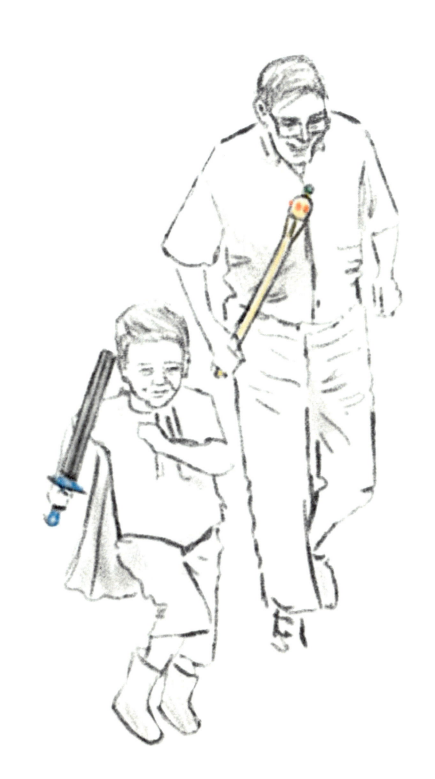

Something has changed about Grandpa now. I can see it in his eyes.
He seems a little sad, but I can't figure out why.

When I ask to play our favorite game - he lets out a little sigh.
While we play, Grandpa forgets the rules that he always knew.
He can't even guess when I give him a really BIG clue.

Yesterday, Grandpa could not even remember my sister's name.
That was the very first time I ever saw him cry.
There is something different about Grandpa.
He just doesn't seem the same.

The way he talks and the way he walks is changing day by day.
I know something is wrong with Grandpa. I feel it deep down inside.
I'm going to ask my mom because she would never lie.

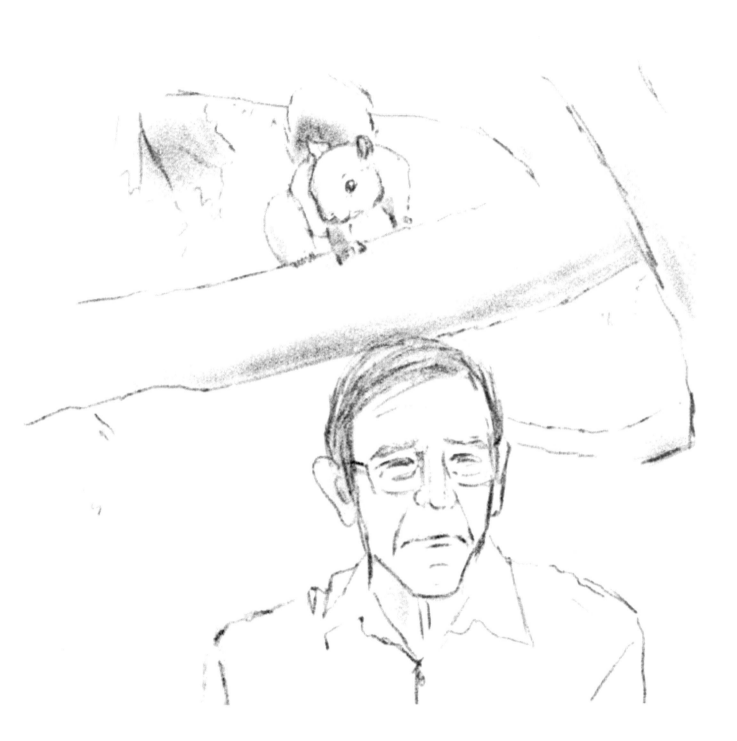

Mom explains that the things I am feeling are not wrong. She says it's our turn to take care of Grandpa and she knows that I'll be strong. Mom says, "Grandpa has something called Lewy Body dementia and it will never go away." We decide to call it Lewy because that is easier to say.

Lewy will cause Grandpa to act or move differently and forget some things that he already knew. She gives me a big hug and tells me, "The only thing I know for sure is that it will never change how he feels about you."

I want to hear what mom has to say, but I really need to know if Grandpa will be okay. Mom tells me that Grandpa will have some pretty hard days and other days will be good. She tells me, "Lewy can seem scary and sometimes funny too, but whatever Grandpa is facing our love will help him through." I don't know why Grandpa got Lewy. It makes me really upset. It is not fair that a sickness can make his brain forget.

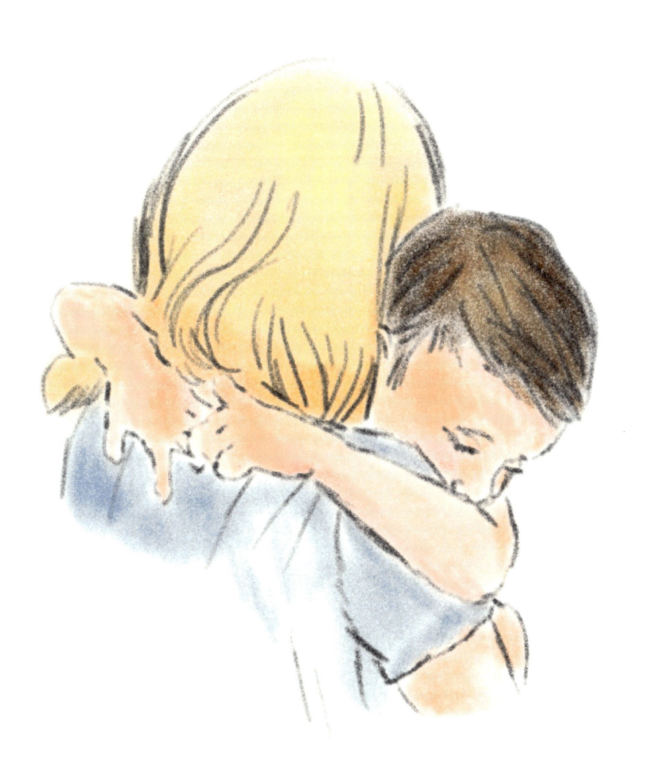

Lewy is like a squirrel, silly as can be -
balancing carefully on branches or hiding in his tree.
Sometimes we hear him scurrying about in the night,
but mostly he spends his days gathering acorns
and hiding them out of sight.

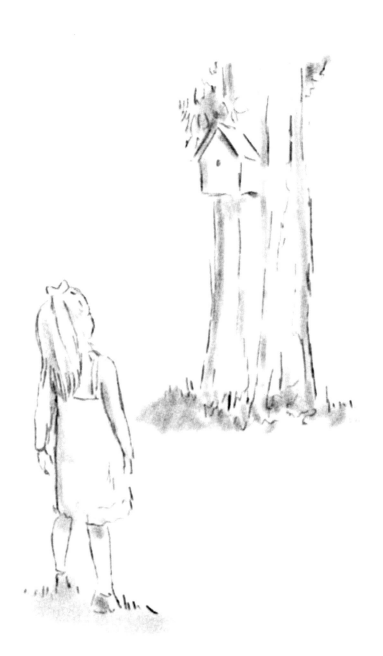

He stays busy doing squirrelly things and hurrying all about.
Quickly darting from one tree to the next, dodging branches and
working hard to keep his acorns from

                      falling

                              to

                                    the

                                          ground.

We never know what to expect when Lewy comes around.

Lewy tries to be sneaky and play silly tricks. He likes to make Grandpa feel a little nutty, but there is one thing he doesn't understand.

My Grandpa has been around a long time and he is a very smart man!

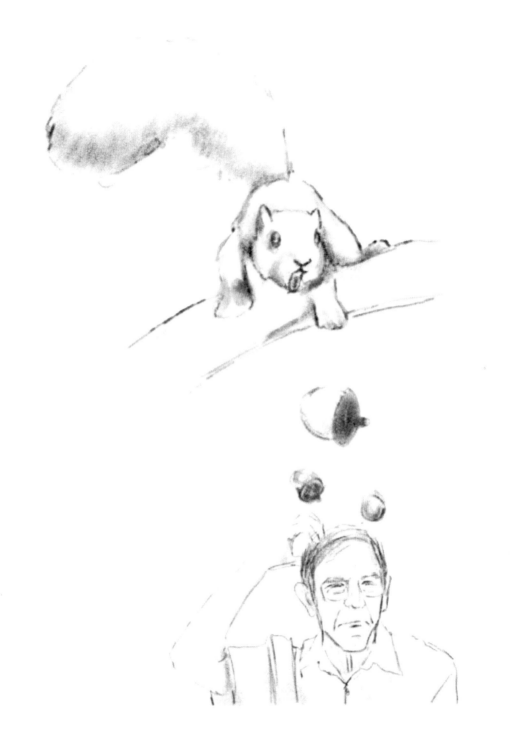

Like Lewy gathering acorns to prepare for snowy days ahead,
Grandpa is pretty clever and his ideas are pretty rad.
Grandpa has been busy planning for hard days to come
and decided to plant a special tree to help both of us
remember the love he feels for me.

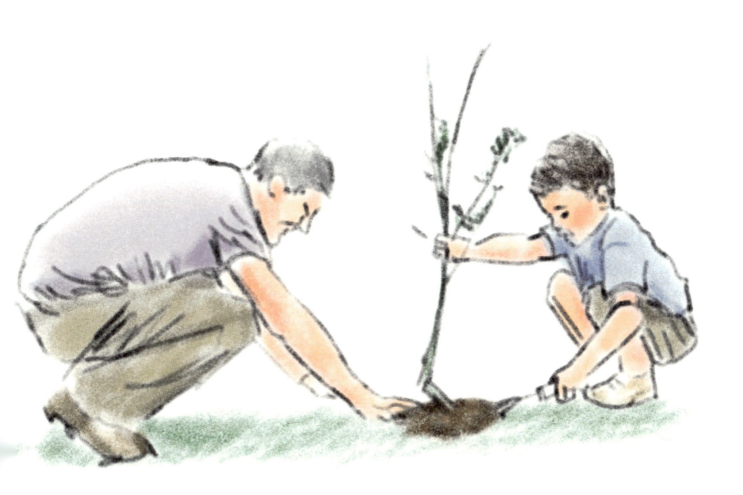

Ever since Lewy came to town, it feels like a roller coaster
with twists and turns and lots of ups and downs.
Things are very different when Lewy is around.

When Lewy shows up, it's hard for Grandpa to remember.
When Lewy stops by, Grandpa moves a bit slower.
When Lewy visits, Grandpa doesn't seem the same.
When Lewy comes around, things get hard and *I* feel sad.

Grandpa, where have you gone? *I* know that you are there.
There must be ways to help you remember how much *I* care.

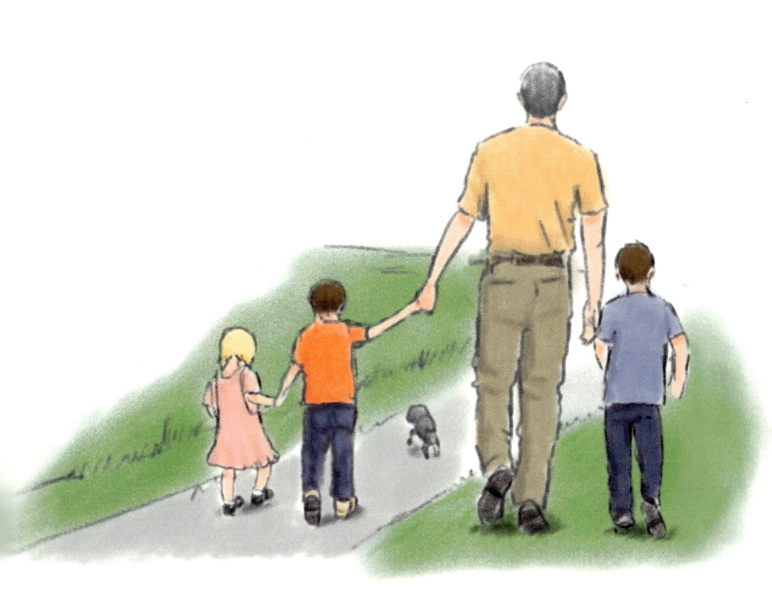

Grandpa, when the earth moves beneath your feet.
I will hold your hand and make your steps complete.
We will dance together and laugh and sing.
For you, I will do anything.

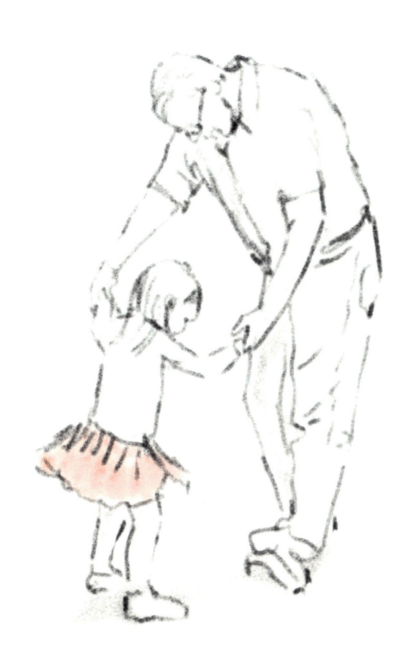

From little seeds grow mighty trees.
Grandpa, please just tell me what you need.
When your body gets tired, I will let you rest.
When your hands shake and it is hard to move,
I will encourage you to try your best.
I'll stand with you if you freeze and feel stuck.
I will help you get through this no matter what.

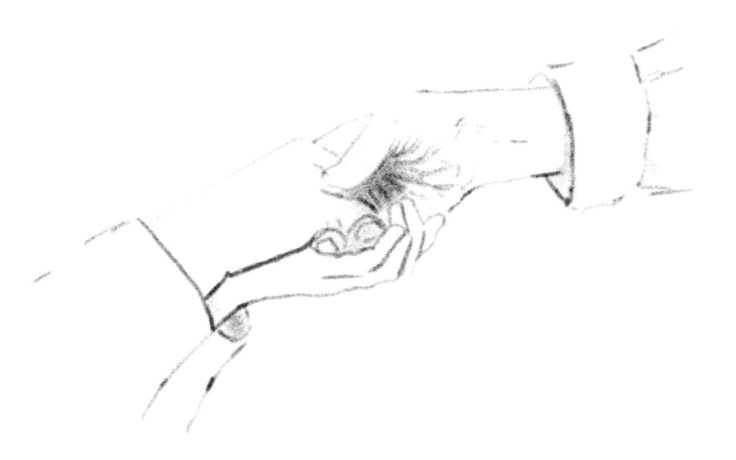

When the sun goes down and things don't make sense.
When the dreams you're dreaming come to life.
When you see something that doesn't feel right.
I will be your light.
Grandpa, there is nothing I can't do.
It is my turn to fight the monsters and be brave for you.

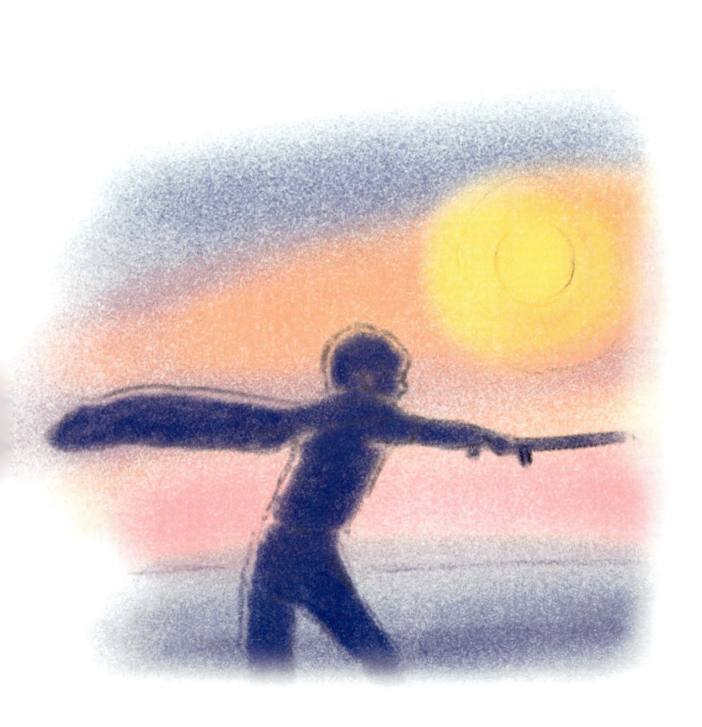

Grandpa, I will help you see this through.
I will help you remember the good dreams.
I will tell you a joke and make things bright.
When your dreams seem so real, I will calm your fears
like you have always done for me at night.

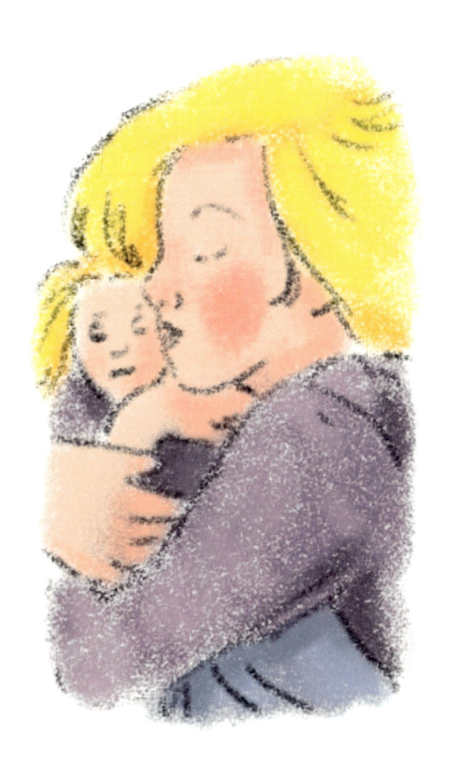

When you forget your words,
I will help you find them.
When your faith is tested,
I will tell you the story of the little acorn who was
destined to become something great.
I will remind you of the mighty oak tree
that stood tall when the winds blew strong.
I will never let you forget your greatness,
like you've done for me all along.

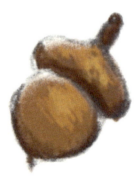

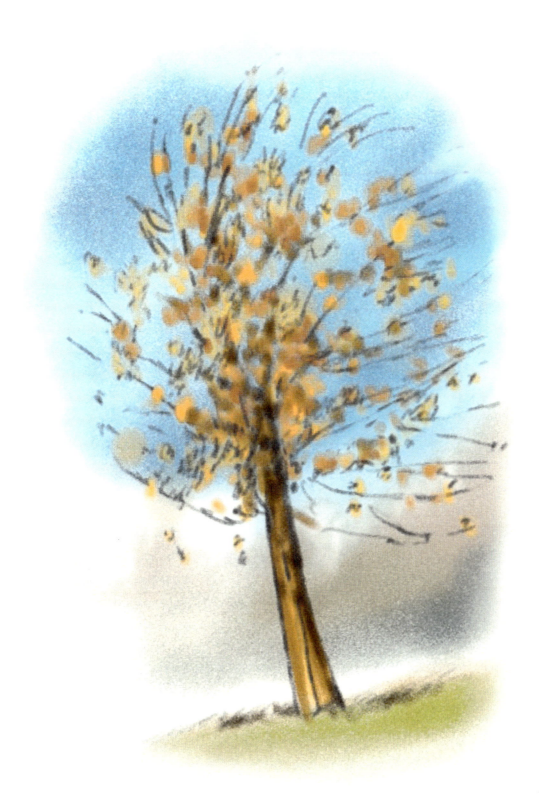

We will pretend and play the way we always have.
You will still be the superhero who saves the day.
Love is our superpower and Lewy can't take that away.
We will imagine the clouds are big pirate ships sailing out to sea.
Heading far beyond the trees - somewhere that sneaky squirrel will never be.

That will be our special place where Lewy cannot go.
Like a safe harbor in the storm; a place that only we know.

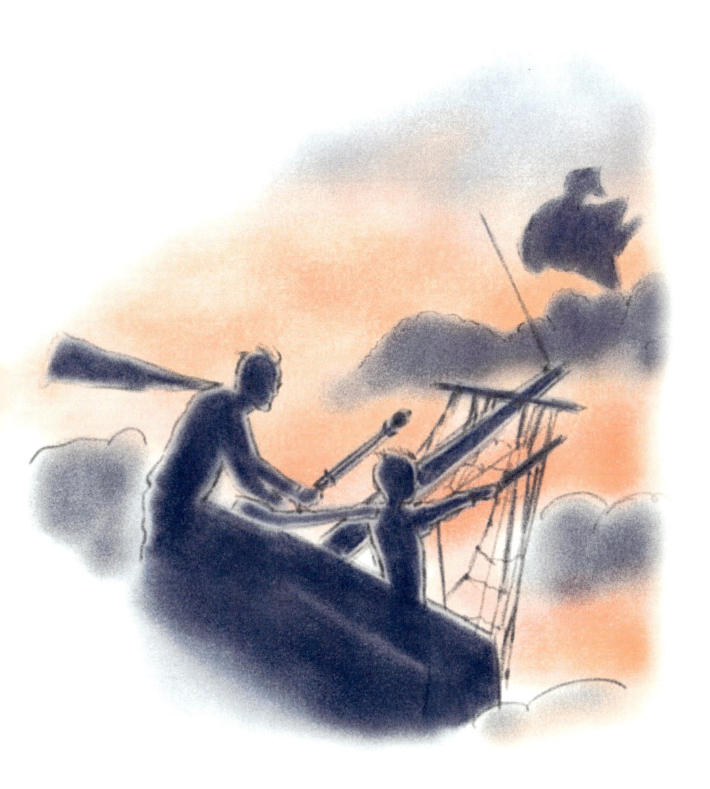

No matter what changes may come our way, together is where we will stay. Our hearts will hold your memories dear. In our hearts your mood is always happy, your movement is always easy and your thoughts are always clear.

My heart song will beat you a rhythm so strong that your feet will have to move along.

If they shuffle mine will too, but if they run I'll be right beside you. We will navigate the path of least resistance.

Working hard to keep Lewy at a distance.

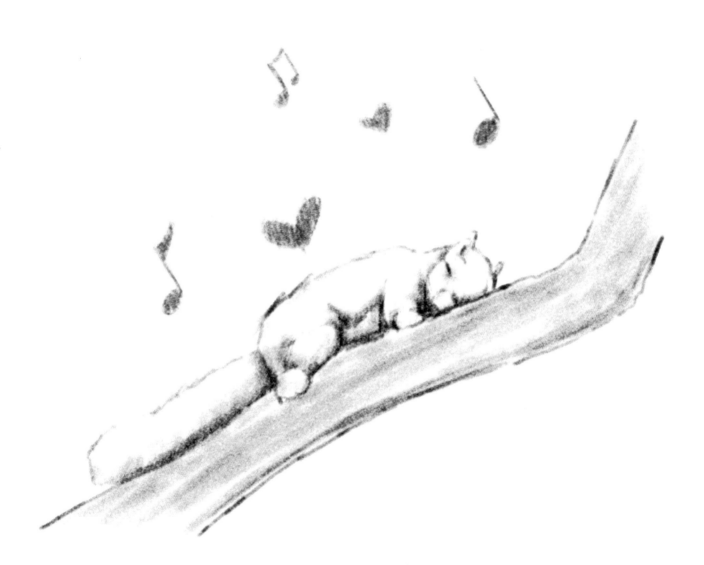

Grandpa looks and acts different now.
Grandpa forgets. He gets upset.
He really doesn't seem like his old self somehow,
but then *I* see it.

That light in his eyes, he remembers!
When he remembers he always tells me that he loves me.
He tells me that he is still my grandpa - my best friend.
He promises that love is one thing Lewy can not change
and that our love will never end.

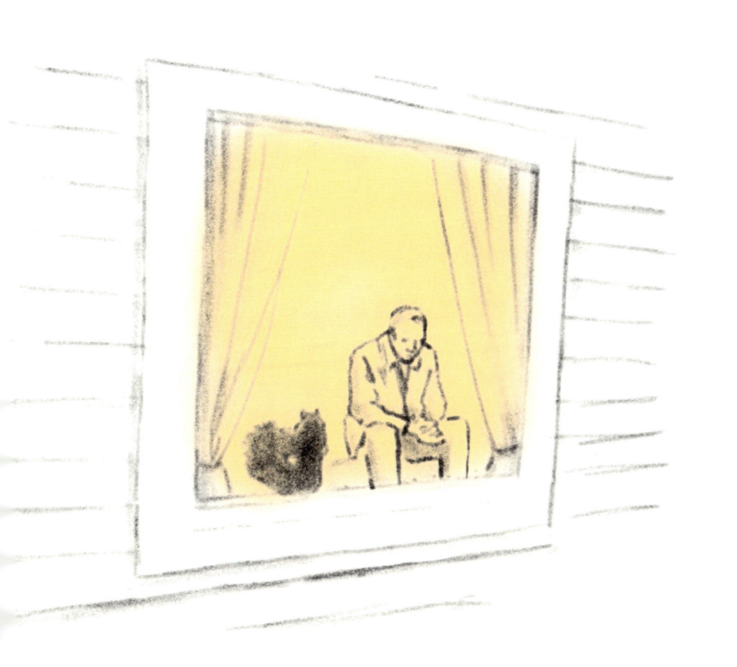

I make a promise to Grandpa too.
I promise to love him through it all.
All of the changes, both big and small
And if there comes a day that we can't be together—

I promise to keep Grandpa in my heart forever.

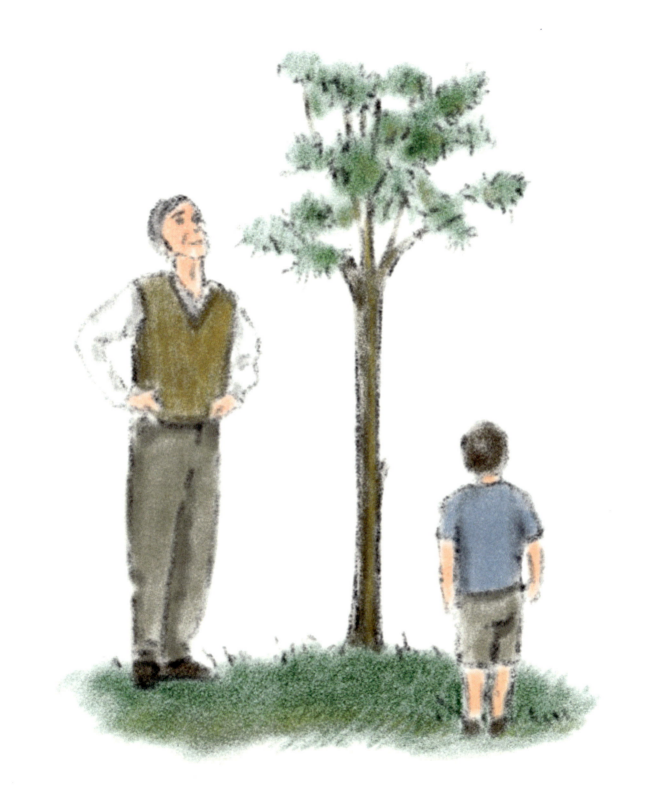

Even though Lewy thinks his sneaky tricks can slow me down.
My journey does not end
because I know that Grandpa's love
has taken root and made me who I am.

I'm growing fast from a seedling to a tree.
Like that little acorn transformed
into a great oak
standing tall and strong,
majestic in its glory.
I, too, am capable of great things--
just by sharing my story.

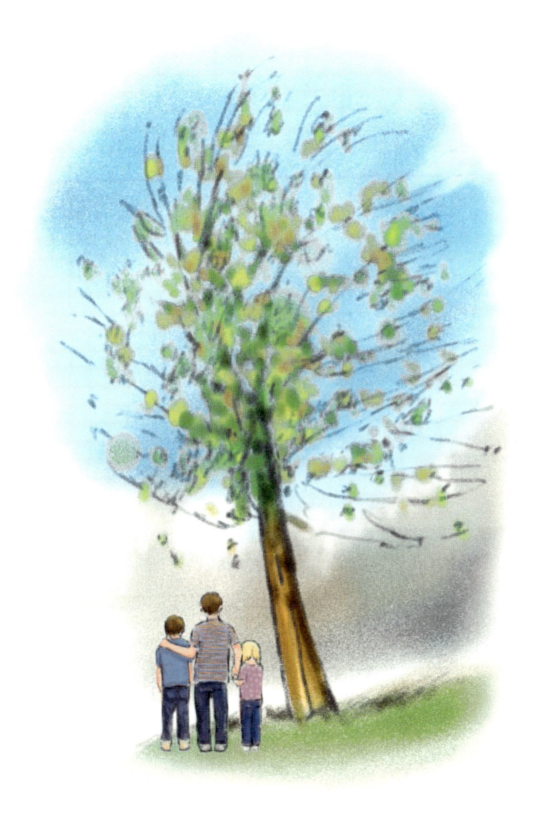

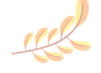

Ways to help your child cope:

Physical and behavior changes from Lewy can be frightening for a child. Give them permission to love from a distance when they need to.

Set the example. Children learn what they live. Your actions and relationship with Lewy will leave a lasting impression on your child. The physical and behavioral changes from LBD can be both frustrating and frightening. When Lewy comes around things will get hard. Always try to act with kindness and compassion.

Changes may be subtle at first, but children are very perceptive. Start a dialogue about the changes that are happening and what can be expected early on. Allow them to ask questions. Keep the answers honest, but general and age appropriate.

Symptoms are not static. When you recognize that it is a "good day" encourage interaction and bonding activities. Have the child read to their loved one, imaginary play or look through family photo albums.

Help your child identify ways they are comfortable helping a loved one. For some children it will be easier to paint a picture or make craft to show their love. Other children are much more hands on and want to help and interact with the loved one. Each child handles change differently, but compassion is displayed in many forms.

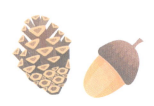

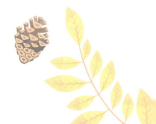

Look for the blessings. It sounds so cliché, but even the darkest times we can find a blessing. Teach your child to look for the rainbow after the storm. Lewy will bring challenges, hardships and tears. It can also bring some beautiful things into your life. The tough times bring special people into our lives or bring us closer to each other.   There were little blessings along our journey through Lewy. They would have been easy to miss if we were so consumed by the storm that we couldn't see the rainbows.

Look for the humor. There is no doubt Lewy is nothing to laugh about, but I do believe you have to find the humor in hard things too. My dad did some silly things. Sometimes we didn't know whether to laugh or cry and other times we got a big belly laugh. Those laughs are the memories we hold onto today.

Get help…if you are a primary caregiver to someone with LBD and trying to raise a child, welcome to the sandwich generation--those struggling to balance caring for children and aging parents at the same time. That's a big order to fill. The demand can be mentally and physically exhausting. Look for resources: support groups, awareness events and respite care to avoid caregiver burnout.

Resources

Lewy Body Dementia Association
912 Killian Hill Road S.W.
Lilburn, GA 30047
website: LBDA.org

LBDA Forum — forum@lbda.org

LBD Caregiver Link
800-LEWYSOS
800-539-9767

Follow us:

Instagram @ grandpaandlewy
Facebook @ Grandpa & Lewy
www.thejollyauthor.com

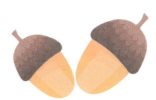

Made in the USA
Middletown, DE
02 November 2021

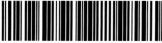